10 WEEKS TO WOW! - ALL ABOUT Y

ABOUT ME: Write down the things I like, What makes

GOALS: What are my goals... What motivates me?

WHY? Write down why I want to make changes in my life!

RELAX: What shall I be doing to relax and unwind?

PLAN: Make a food plan and get organised:

Create Your Own Food Library and Set Menus - (Back Pages) - See online Videos for Set Up Examples...

Author: Jonathan Bowers
All rights reserved. No part of this work may be reproduced or utilised in any form or by means of electronic or mechanical, including photocopying, recording or by any information storage or retrieval system, without the prior written permission of the author. The author nor The Body Plan Plus take responsibility for any possible consequences from any procedure, exercise or action by any persons reading or using the following information in this Diet Diary. (2017) This diary is compatible with Weight Watchers TM Plans. It is not an official diary, no copy written words have been used ensuring the protection of the original plan formula.

10 WEEKS TO WOW! - ONLINE EXTRA CONTENT

There just isn't enough space for it all…!

All the pages that can't fit in this Food Diary can be found on my Website.

www.thebodyplanplus.com

It's an education and everything I learnt. This knowledge made my 7 Stone Weight Loss Journey a success. I urge you to read it and learn it because it will make you look at weight loss and exercise differently. Motivation to lose weight is one thing, but motivation and knowledge makes it a whole lot easier.

If you would like to read about my Journey, simply visit my website and choose **>** About Me

If you have any questions, please don't hesitate to get in touch…

Tania Carter x

Find the Missing Pages.

To find the online extra content (10 Weeks to Wow!) Go to my site and select **> More**

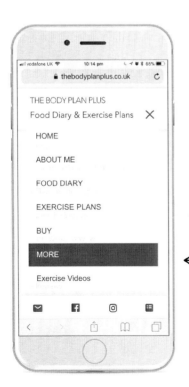

In this section you will find:

- Calorie Goal Calculator
- The Missing Pages (TheBody Plan Plus)
- Exercise Videos
- 10 Weeks to Wow!
- Home Workout Equipment
- Exercise Videos
- Calories Per Gram Calculator
- Quick View Calorie Library
- Easy Set Menus

WEIGHT TRACKER GRAPH

Enter your "**Stone**" Weight only in **Box A** - then mark on the graph your "**Pound**" Weight!

HOW MUCH AND HOW FAST?

You are looking to lose a healthy 1 to 1 and a half pound per week. Any more than this and your body may go into starvation mode. You want to avoid this at all costs because this may result in failure, or your weight coming back **super fast** as soon as your diet cycle ends. To avoid this and ensure success go to our help page for more information and how to avoid this situation. "Success is yours with a little knowledge"

Visit: www.thebodyplanplus.com
From the Home Page, select **>** More - then **>** 10 Weeks to Wow!

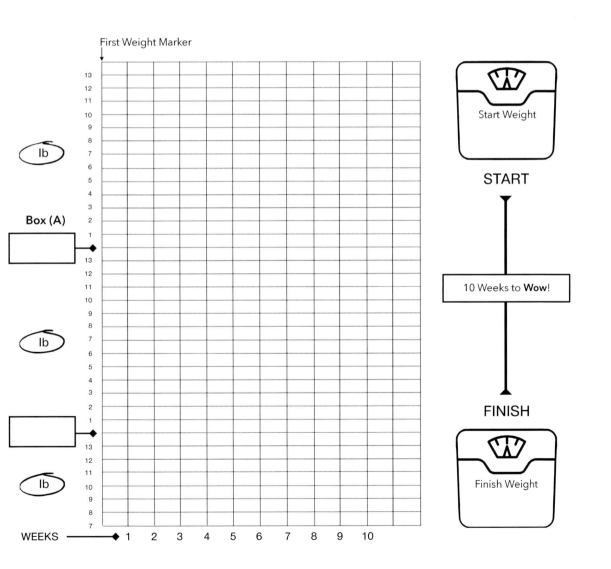

TICKS AND BEVERAGES

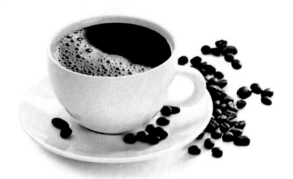

Your beverages are just as important as your meals. Lots of people who are on a diet forget that beverages contain Calories. Some people drink more beverages than others. Sometimes this may be a work environment factor or simply drinking becomes a habit rather than a need.

"Counting ticks is like counting Calories"

If we all took in fluids for our needs only, we would only drink water. This would be a good thing, but we don't simply drink to nourish and hydrate our bodies anymore, we drink for flavour, enjoyment and to socialise.

Beverages taste nice and supply us with a little boost or kick we are looking for.
The most common beverages are, you guessed it, tea, coffee and hot chocolate.

☕ + 1 Sugar = 30 Calories x 10 Cups = **300 Calories**

The reason you need to place a tick on your Diary page each time you have a beverage, is so you can see at a glance how many beverages you are having!

You may be shocked at the amount you do have. Reducing your beverages alone may be all the difference you're looking for to lose weight.

Simply looking at the number of ticks on your page may give you a true picture to whether you are just having too many, or too many in one particular part of the day. You may be able to say to yourself - NO more coffees in the morning, or I will at least reduce this by half!

If you take sugar with your Tea & Coffee, we have a clever little way for you to reduce this by half, or to nothing without you evening noticing it.   Visit our website for more information.

YOUR BODY PLAN EXERCISE ROUTINE

Exercising is optional, but advised… It's easier to burn Calories off than starve them off! This is a simple exercise formula and has be designed to cater for all levels of fitness, stamina and flexibility, it works brilliantly because you get to choose the exercises that are right for
you and your body type.

Perform your exercises and tick completed on your planner page to keep a record of your progress throughout the forthcoming weeks.

This exercise programme is - Timed Exercise and Timed Resting. Perform your exercises for **60 Seconds** and rest for **60 Seconds**. To increase the intensity of your routine, you can reduce your resting times
by **15 to 30 Seconds**.

Perform your chosen exercises for **60 Seconds** and Rest / Pause for **60 Seconds**. Repeat each exercise **3 times in a row**. Tick when completed so you can track your performance.

Low Level Intensity
- ✓ Chair Squats
- ✓ The Bridge
- ✓ Quater Squats
- ✓ The Plank

Medium Level Intensity
- ✓ Air Punches
- ✓ Free Squats
- ✓ Lunges
- ✓ Stair Walking

High Level Intensity
- ✓ Jumping Jacks
- ✓ Burpees
- ✓ Mountain Climbers
- ✓ Walking Lunges

A walk through Exercise Video can be found for each Exercise on my website: www.thebodyplanplus.com While you're visiting, check out my amazing weight loss exercise formulas for all levels of fitness and **Weight Loss Goals**.

From the Home Page select **> More**, then **> 10 Weeks to Wow**"

ONLINE CALORIE GOAL CALCULATOR

When you are ready to get your ideal Calorie Goal - Go to my website and select
> MORE and then select **> Calorie Goal Calculator**. Enter your information as required: **Gender - Age - Weight - Height - Exercise Level**

Be honest about your Exercise (**PART 3**) as this may impact your results. Saying you do more **Exercise** than you actually do will result in more Calories being added to your total.

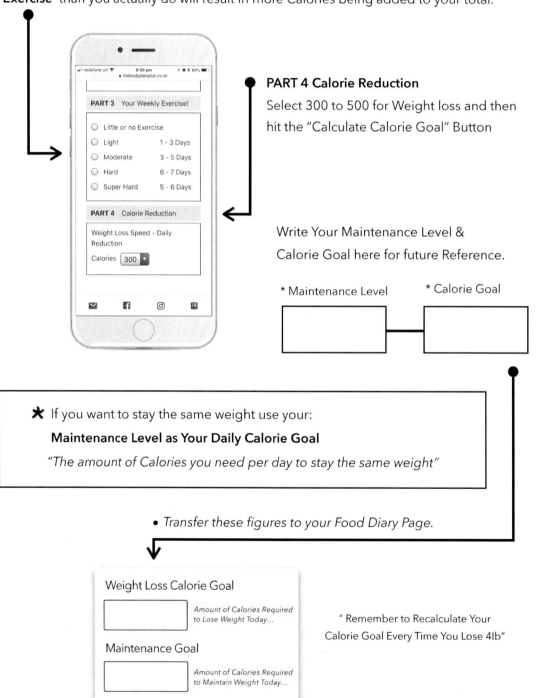

PART 4 Calorie Reduction
Select 300 to 500 for Weight loss and then hit the "Calculate Calorie Goal" Button

Write Your Maintenance Level &
Calorie Goal here for future Reference.

* Maintenance Level   * Calorie Goal

★ If you want to stay the same weight use your:
   Maintenance Level as Your Daily Calorie Goal
   "The amount of Calories you need per day to stay the same weight"

• *Transfer these figures to your Food Diary Page.*

Weight Loss Calorie Goal
Amount of Calories Required to Lose Weight Today...

Maintenance Goal
Amount of Calories Required to Maintain Weight Today...

" Remember to Recalculate Your Calorie Goal Every Time You Lose 4lb"

CALORIES PER GRAM CALCULATOR

To make life easy the Calorie Value should be a single unit, then it becomes easy to work everything out.

Example: If your Ham slices are 120 Calories "**Per 100 Grams**" and your Portion weighed 50 Grams - How many Calories are in your Portion? The Calculation would be: 120 divided by 100 x 50 = 60 Calories.

Once again you don't have to do any Calculations…. All you have to do is use my Online Calculator. Go to my website - Select **> More** and then - Calories Per Gram Calculator ⟶

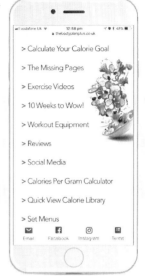

Example: Ham

Calories Per Gram Calculator

Calories (kcal) Per 100 Grams	120
Portion Weight in Grams	50
Calculate	
Calories Per Gram =	1.2
Calories in Your Portion =	60

VERY CLEVER!

1. Enter the Calories Per 100 Gram.

2. Enter the Portion Weight in Grams.
   Either your own Scale Weight - Or Packet Weight.

3. Hit Calculate.
   Record the information in your Calorie Library for future reference.

TIME SAVING TIP

When you have found the Calories Per Gram Calculator on your Mobile Device. Add the Page to your Home Screen. A small icon will appear on your phone which will allow you to open the Calculator straight away as and when you need it.

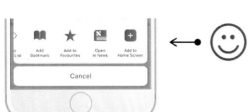

VIDEO DEMO

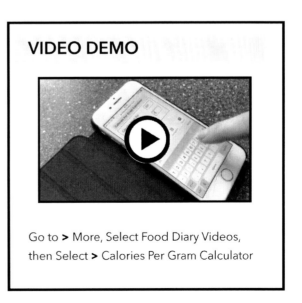

Go to **>** More, Select Food Diary Videos, then Select **>** Calories Per Gram Calculator

DATE: / /   Bed [:]   Awake [:]   Hours [ ]

NOTES

TO DO
- [ ]
- [ ]
- [ ]
- [ ]
- [ ]

Today I am grateful for:

MEAL PLANNER - Tomorrows Meals Organised!

TODAYS HEALTHY HABITS - Five a day - Colour me in - Water - Fruit & Veggies

ACTIVITY

Total Steps [ ]

Total Floors / Flights [ ]

EXERCISE

Completed Exercise Routine

3 x 1 Min / Exercise 1

3 x 1 Min / Exercise 2

3 x 1 Min / Exercise 3

Calorie / Points Total

[ ]   (A) + (B) + (C) ←

Beverage Total

[ ] ✓

Weight Loss Calorie Goal

[ ]   *Amount of Calories Required to Lose Weight Today...*

Maintenance Goal

[ ]   *Amount of Calories Required to Maintain Weight Today...*

BREAKFAST / MORNING

Calories / Points ✓

LUNCH / AFTERNOON

DINNER / EVENING

Morning: Calories / Points
A

Afternoon: Calories / Points
B

Evening: Calories / Points
C

DATE: / /   Bed :   Awake :   Hours

NOTES
TO DO

Today I am grateful for:

MEAL PLANNER - Tomorrows Meals Organised!

TODAYS HEALTHY HABITS - Five a day - Colour me in - Water - Fruit & Veggies

ACTIVITY

Total Steps

Total Floors / Flights

EXERCISE

Completed Exercise Routine

3 x 1 Min / Exercise 1

3 x 1 Min / Exercise 2

3 x 1 Min / Exercise 3

Calorie / Points Total

(A) + (B) + (C)

Beverage Total

Weight Loss Calorie Goal

Amount of Calories Required to Lose Weight Today...

Maintenance Goal

Amount of Calories Required to Maintain Weight Today...

BREAKFAST / MORNING

Calories / Points

LUNCH / AFTERNOON

DINNER / EVENING

Morning: Calories / Points **A**

Afternoon: Calories / Points **B**

Evening: Calories / Points **C**

DATE: / /   Bed ☐ : ☐   Awake ☐ : ☐   Hours ☐

NOTES

TO DO
☐
☐
☐
☐
Today I am grateful for: ☐

MEAL PLANNER - Tomorrows Meals Organised!

TODAYS HEALTHY HABITS - Five a day - Colour me in - Water - Fruit & Veggies

ACTIVITY

Total Steps ☐

Total Floors / Flights ☐

EXERCISE

Completed Exercise Routine

3 x 1 Min / Exercise 1 ☐☐☐

3 x 1 Min / Exercise 2 ☐☐☐

3 x 1 Min / Exercise 3 ☐☐☐

Calorie / Points Total

☐ (A) + (B) + (C)

Beverage Total

☐ ✓

Weight Loss Calorie Goal

☐ *Amount of Calories Required to Lose Weight Today...*

Maintenance Goal

☐ *Amount of Calories Required to Maintain Weight Today...*

BREAKFAST / MORNING

Calories / Points ✓

LUNCH / AFTERNOON

DINNER / EVENING

Morning: Calories / Points
A

Afternoon: Calories / Points
B

Evening: Calories / Points
C

DATE: / /   Bed ☐ : ☐   Awake ☐ : ☐   Hours ☐

NOTES

TO DO

Today I am grateful for:

MEAL PLANNER - Tomorrows Meals Organised!

TODAYS HEALTHY HABITS - Five a day - Colour me in - Water - Fruit & Veggies

ACTIVITY

Total Steps ☐

Total Floors / Flights ☐

EXERCISE

Completed Exercise Routine

3 x 1 Min / Exercise 1

3 x 1 Min / Exercise 2

3 x 1 Min / Exercise 3

Calorie / Points Total

☐   (A) + (B) + (C) ←

Beverage Total

☐ ✓

Weight Loss Calorie Goal

☐   *Amount of Calories Required to Lose Weight Today...*

Maintenance Goal

☐   *Amount of Calories Required to Maintain Weight Today...*

BREAKFAST / MORNING

Calories / Points ✓

LUNCH / AFTERNOON

DINNER / EVENING

Morning: Calories / Points **A**

Afternoon: Calories / Points **B**

Evening: Calories / Points **C**

DATE: /   /   Bed [:]   Awake [:]   Hours [   ]

NOTES

TO DO

Today I am grateful for:

MEAL PLANNER - Tomorrows Meals Organised!

TODAYS HEALTHY HABITS - Five a day - Colour me in - Water - Fruit & Veggies

ACTIVITY

Total Steps

Total Floors / Flights

Calorie / Points Total

(A) + (B) + (C)

Beverage Total

EXERCISE

Completed Exercise Routine

3 x 1 Min / Exercise 1

3 x 1 Min / Exercise 2

3 x 1 Min / Exercise 3

Weight Loss Calorie Goal

Amount of Calories Required to Lose Weight Today...

Maintenance Goal

Amount of Calories Required to Maintain Weight Today...

BREAKFAST / MORNING

Calories / Points

LUNCH / AFTERNOON

DINNER / EVENING

Morning: Calories / Points   Afternoon: Calories / Points   Evening: Calories / Points

A   **B**   **C**

DATE: / /   Bed ☐ : ☐   Awake ☐ : ☐   Hours ☐

NOTES

TO DO
☐
☐
☐
☐

Today I am grateful for: ☐

MEAL PLANNER - Tomorrows Meals Organised!

TODAYS HEALTHY HABITS - Five a day - Colour me in - Water - Fruit & Veggies

ACTIVITY

Total Steps ☐

Total Floors / Flights ☐

EXERCISE

Completed Exercise Routine

3 x 1 Min / Exercise 1 ☐ ☐ ☐

3 x 1 Min / Exercise 2 ☐ ☐ ☐

3 x 1 Min / Exercise 3 ☐ ☐ ☐

Calorie / Points Total

☐   (A) + (B) + (C) ←

Beverage Total

☐ ✓

Weight Loss Calorie Goal

☐   *Amount of Calories Required to Lose Weight Today...*

Maintenance Goal

☐   *Amount of Calories Required to Maintain Weight Today...*

BREAKFAST / MORNING

Calories / Points ✓

LUNCH / AFTERNOON

DINNER / EVENING

Morning: Calories / Points **A**

Afternoon: Calories / Points **B**

Evening: Calories / Points **C**

DATE: /   /   Bed :   Awake :   Hours

NOTES

TO DO

Today I am grateful for:

MEAL PLANNER - Tomorrows Meals Organised!

TODAYS HEALTHY HABITS - Five a day - Colour me in - Water - Fruit & Veggies

ACTIVITY

Total Steps

Total Floors / Flights

EXERCISE

Completed Exercise Routine

3 x 1 Min / Exercise 1

3 x 1 Min / Exercise 2

3 x 1 Min / Exercise 3

Calorie / Points Total

(A) + (B) + (C)

Beverage Total

Weight Loss Calorie Goal

Amount of Calories Required to Lose Weight Today...

Maintenance Goal

Amount of Calories Required to Maintain Weight Today...

BREAKFAST / MORNING

Calories / Points ✓

LUNCH / AFTERNOON

DINNER / EVENING

Morning: Calories / Points **A**

Afternoon: Calories / Points **B**

Evening: Calories / Points **C**

DATE: / /   Bed :   Awake :   Hours

NOTES

TO DO

Today I am grateful for:

MEAL PLANNER - Tomorrows Meals Organised!

TODAYS HEALTHY HABITS - Five a day - Colour me in - Water - Fruit & Veggies

ACTIVITY

Total Steps

Total Floors / Flights

EXERCISE

Completed Exercise Routine

3 x 1 Min / Exercise 1

3 x 1 Min / Exercise 2

3 x 1 Min / Exercise 3

Calorie / Points Total

(A) + (B) + (C)

Beverage Total

Weight Loss Calorie Goal

Amount of Calories Required to Lose Weight Today...

Maintenance Goal

Amount of Calories Required to Maintain Weight Today...

BREAKFAST / MORNING

Calories / Points ✓

LUNCH / AFTERNOON

DINNER / EVENING

Morning: Calories / Points
A

Afternoon: Calories / Points
B

Evening: Calories / Points
C

DATE: /   /   Bed [:]   Awake [:]   Hours [   ]

NOTES

TO DO

Today I am grateful for:

MEAL PLANNER - Tomorrows Meals Organised!

TODAYS HEALTHY HABITS - Five a day - Colour me in - Water - Fruit & Veggies

ACTIVITY

Total Steps [   ]

Total Floors / Flights [   ]

EXERCISE

Completed Exercise Routine

3 x 1 Min / Exercise 1

3 x 1 Min / Exercise 2

3 x 1 Min / Exercise 3

Calorie / Points Total

[   ]   (A) + (B) + (C) ←

Beverage Total

[   ]

Weight Loss Calorie Goal

[   ]   *Amount of Calories Required to Lose Weight Today...*

Maintenance Goal

[   ]   *Amount of Calories Required to Maintain Weight Today...*

BREAKFAST / MORNING

Calories / Points ✓

LUNCH / AFTERNOON

DINNER / EVENING

Morning: Calories / Points   Afternoon: Calories / Points   Evening: Calories / Points

A ☐   **B** ☐   **C** ☐

DATE: / / **Bed** : **Awake** : **Hours**

NOTES   TO DO

Today I am grateful for:

MEAL PLANNER - Tomorrows Meals Organised!

TODAYS HEALTHY HABITS - Five a day - Colour me in - Water - Fruit & Veggies

ACTIVITY

Total Steps

Total Floors / Flights

EXERCISE

Completed Exercise Routine

3 x 1 Min / Exercise 1

3 x 1 Min / Exercise 2

3 x 1 Min / Exercise 3

Calorie / Points Total

(A) + (B) + (C)

Beverage Total

Weight Loss Calorie Goal

Amount of Calories Required to Lose Weight Today...

Maintenance Goal

Amount of Calories Required to Maintain Weight Today...

BREAKFAST / MORNING

Calories / Points

LUNCH / AFTERNOON

DINNER / EVENING

Morning: Calories / Points **A**

Afternoon: Calories / Points **B**

Evening: Calories / Points **C**

DATE: / / Bed : Awake : Hours

NOTES

TO DO

Today I am grateful for:

MEAL PLANNER - Tomorrows Meals Organised!

TODAYS HEALTHY HABITS - Five a day - Colour me in - Water - Fruit & Veggies

ACTIVITY

Total Steps

Total Floors / Flights

Calorie / Points Total

(A) + (B) + (C)

Beverage Total

EXERCISE

Completed Exercise Routine

3 x 1 Min / Exercise 1

3 x 1 Min / Exercise 2

3 x 1 Min / Exercise 3

Weight Loss Calorie Goal

Amount of Calories Required to Lose Weight Today...

Maintenance Goal

Amount of Calories Required to Maintain Weight Today...

BREAKFAST / MORNING

Calories / Points

LUNCH / AFTERNOON

DINNER / EVENING

Morning: Calories / Points **A**

Afternoon: Calories / Points **B**

Evening: Calories / Points **C**

DATE: /   /   Bed :   Awake :   Hours

NOTES

TO DO

Today I am grateful for:

MEAL PLANNER - Tomorrows Meals Organised!

TODAYS HEALTHY HABITS - Five a day - Colour me in - Water - Fruit & Veggies

ACTIVITY

Total Steps

Total Floors / Flights

EXERCISE

Completed Exercise Routine

3 x 1 Min / Exercise 1

3 x 1 Min / Exercise 2

3 x 1 Min / Exercise 3

Calorie / Points Total

(A) + (B) + (C)

Beverage Total

Weight Loss Calorie Goal

Amount of Calories Required to Lose Weight Today...

Maintenance Goal

Amount of Calories Required to Maintain Weight Today...

BREAKFAST / MORNING

Calories / Points

LUNCH / AFTERNOON

DINNER / EVENING

Morning: Calories / Points
A

Afternoon: Calories / Points
B

Evening: Calories / Points
C

DATE: / / **Bed** : **Awake** : **Hours**

NOTES

TO DO

Today I am grateful for:

MEAL PLANNER - Tomorrows Meals Organised!

TODAYS HEALTHY HABITS - Five a day - Colour me in - Water - Fruit & Veggies

ACTIVITY

Total Steps

Total Floors / Flights

EXERCISE

Completed Exercise Routine

3 x 1 Min / Exercise 1

3 x 1 Min / Exercise 2

3 x 1 Min / Exercise 3

Calorie / Points Total

(A) + (B) + (C)

Beverage Total

Weight Loss Calorie Goal

Amount of Calories Required to Lose Weight Today...

Maintenance Goal

Amount of Calories Required to Maintain Weight Today...

BREAKFAST / MORNING

Calories / Points

LUNCH / AFTERNOON

DINNER / EVENING

Morning: Calories / Points **A**

Afternoon: Calories / Points **B**

Evening: Calories / Points **C**

DATE: /   /   Bed [:   ]   Awake [:   ]   Hours [   ]

NOTES

TO DO

Today I am grateful for:

MEAL PLANNER - Tomorrows Meals Organised!

TODAYS HEALTHY HABITS - Five a day - Colour me in - Water - Fruit & Veggies

ACTIVITY

Total Steps

Total Floors / Flights

Calorie / Points Total

(A) + (B) + (C)

Beverage Total

EXERCISE

Completed Exercise Routine

3 x 1 Min / Exercise 1

3 x 1 Min / Exercise 2

3 x 1 Min / Exercise 3

Weight Loss Calorie Goal

Amount of Calories Required to Lose Weight Today...

Maintenance Goal

Amount of Calories Required to Maintain Weight Today...

BREAKFAST / MORNING

Calories / Points

LUNCH / AFTERNOON

DINNER / EVENING

Morning: Calories / Points **A**

Afternoon: Calories / Points **B**

Evening: Calories / Points **C**

DATE: /   /   Bed [:]   Awake [:]   Hours [   ]

NOTES   TO DO

☐
☐
☐
☐

Today I am grateful for: ☐

MEAL PLANNER - Tomorrows Meals Organised!

TODAYS HEALTHY HABITS - Five a day - Colour me in - Water - Fruit & Veggies

ACTIVITY

Total Steps [   ]

Total Floors / Flights [   ]

EXERCISE

Completed Exercise Routine

3 x 1 Min / Exercise 1   ☐ ☐ ☐

3 x 1 Min / Exercise 2   ☐ ☐ ☐

3 x 1 Min / Exercise 3   ☐ ☐ ☐

Calorie / Points Total

[   ]   (A) + (B) + (C) ←

Beverage Total

[   ] ✓

Weight Loss Calorie Goal

[   ]   *Amount of Calories Required to Lose Weight Today...*

Maintenance Goal

[   ]   *Amount of Calories Required to Maintain Weight Today...*

BREAKFAST / MORNING

Calories / Points

LUNCH / AFTERNOON

DINNER / EVENING

Morning: Calories / Points

A

Afternoon: Calories / Points

B

Evening: Calories / Points

C

DATE: ___ / ___ / ___   Bed ___:___   Awake ___:___   Hours ___

NOTES

TO DO

Today I am grateful for: _____

MEAL PLANNER - Tomorrows Meals Organised!

TODAYS HEALTHY HABITS - Five a day - Colour me in - Water - Fruit & Veggies

ACTIVITY

Total Steps _____

Total Floors / Flights _____

Calorie / Points Total

_____ (A) + (B) + (C)

Beverage Total

_____

EXERCISE

Completed Exercise Routine

3 x 1 Min / Exercise 1

3 x 1 Min / Exercise 2

3 x 1 Min / Exercise 3

Weight Loss Calorie Goal

_____

Amount of Calories Required to Lose Weight Today...

Maintenance Goal

_____

Amount of Calories Required to Maintain Weight Today...

BREAKFAST / MORNING

Calories / Points

LUNCH / AFTERNOON

DINNER / EVENING

Morning: Calories / Points **A**

Afternoon: Calories / Points **B**

Evening: Calories / Points **C**

DATE: / / Bed : Awake : Hours

NOTES

Today I am grateful for:

TO DO

MEAL PLANNER - Tomorrows Meals Organised!

TODAYS HEALTHY HABITS - Five a day - Colour me in - Water - Fruit & Veggies

ACTIVITY

Total Steps

Total Floors / Flights

EXERCISE

Completed Exercise Routine

3 x 1 Min / Exercise 1

3 x 1 Min / Exercise 2

3 x 1 Min / Exercise 3

Calorie / Points Total

(A) + (B) + (C)

Beverage Total

Weight Loss Calorie Goal

Amount of Calories Required to Lose Weight Today...

Maintenance Goal

Amount of Calories Required to Maintain Weight Today...

BREAKFAST / MORNING

Calories / Points ✓

LUNCH / AFTERNOON

DINNER / EVENING

Morning: Calories / Points — **A**

Afternoon: Calories / Points — **B**

Evening: Calories / Points — **C**

DATE: /   /   Bed [:]   Awake [:]   Hours [   ]

NOTES   TO DO

☐
☐
☐
☐

Today I am grateful for: ☐

MEAL PLANNER - Tomorrows Meals Organised!

TODAYS HEALTHY HABITS - Five a day - Colour me in - Water - Fruit & Veggies

ACTIVITY

Total Steps [   ]

Total Floors / Flights [   ]

EXERCISE

Completed Exercise Routine

3 x 1 Min / Exercise 1   ☐ ☐ ☐

3 x 1 Min / Exercise 2   ☐ ☐ ☐

3 x 1 Min / Exercise 3   ☐ ☐ ☐

Calorie / Points Total

[   ]   (A) + (B) + (C) ←

Beverage Total

[   ] ✓

Weight Loss Calorie Goal

[   ]   *Amount of Calories Required to Lose Weight Today...*

Maintenance Goal

[   ]   *Amount of Calories Required to Maintain Weight Today...*

BREAKFAST / MORNING

Calories / Points

LUNCH / AFTERNOON

DINNER / EVENING

Morning: Calories / Points

A

Afternoon: Calories / Points

B

Evening: Calories / Points

C

DATE: /   /   Bed [:]   Awake [:]   Hours [ ]

NOTES   TO DO

☐
☐
☐
☐
Today I am grateful for: ☐

MEAL PLANNER - Tomorrows Meals Organised!

TODAYS HEALTHY HABITS - Five a day - Colour me in - Water - Fruit & Veggies

ACTIVITY

Total Steps [   ]

Total Floors / Flights [   ]

Calorie / Points Total

[   ] (A) + (B) + (C) ←

Beverage Total

[   ] ✓

EXERCISE

Completed Exercise Routine

3 x 1 Min / Exercise 1   ☐ ☐ ☐

3 x 1 Min / Exercise 2   ☐ ☐ ☐

3 x 1 Min / Exercise 3   ☐ ☐ ☐

Weight Loss Calorie Goal

[   ] *Amount of Calories Required to Lose Weight Today...*

Maintenance Goal

[   ] *Amount of Calories Required to Maintain Weight Today...*

BREAKFAST / MORNING

Calories / Points

LUNCH / AFTERNOON

DINNER / EVENING

Morning: Calories / Points **A**

Afternoon: Calories / Points **B**

Evening: Calories / Points **C**

DATE: ___ / ___ / ___   Bed ☐ : ☐   Awake ☐ : ☐   Hours ☐

NOTES

Today I am grateful for:

TO DO

☐
☐
☐
☐
☐

MEAL PLANNER - Tomorrows Meals Organised!

TODAYS HEALTHY HABITS - Five a day - Colour me in - Water - Fruit & Veggies

ACTIVITY

Total Steps ☐

Total Floors / Flights ☐

EXERCISE

Completed Exercise Routine

3 x 1 Min / Exercise 1   ☐ ☐ ☐
3 x 1 Min / Exercise 2   ☐ ☐ ☐
3 x 1 Min / Exercise 3   ☐ ☐ ☐

Calorie / Points Total

☐   (A) + (B) + (C) ←

Beverage Total

☐ ✓

Weight Loss Calorie Goal

☐   *Amount of Calories Required to Lose Weight Today...*

Maintenance Goal

☐   *Amount of Calories Required to Maintain Weight Today...*

BREAKFAST / MORNING

Calories / Points ✓

LUNCH / AFTERNOON

DINNER / EVENING

Morning: Calories / Points
A

Afternoon: Calories / Points
B

Evening: Calories / Points
C

DATE: ___ / ___ / ___   Bed ___:___   Awake ___:___   Hours ___

NOTES

_____
_____
_____
_____
Today I am grateful for: _____

TO DO

- [ ] _____
- [ ] _____
- [ ] _____
- [ ] _____
- [ ] _____

MEAL PLANNER - Tomorrows Meals Organised!

_____
_____
_____
_____
_____

TODAYS HEALTHY HABITS - Five a day - Colour me in - Water - Fruit & Veggies

ACTIVITY

Total Steps [ ]

Total Floors / Flights [ ]

EXERCISE

Completed Exercise Routine

3 x 1 Min / Exercise 1   [ ][ ][ ]

3 x 1 Min / Exercise 2   [ ][ ][ ]

3 x 1 Min / Exercise 3   [ ][ ][ ]

Calorie / Points Total

[ ]   (A) + (B) + (C)

Beverage Total

[ ] ✓

Weight Loss Calorie Goal

[ ]   *Amount of Calories Required to Lose Weight Today...*

Maintenance Goal

[ ]   *Amount of Calories Required to Maintain Weight Today...*

BREAKFAST / MORNING

Calories / Points

LUNCH / AFTERNOON

DINNER / EVENING

Morning: Calories / Points **A**

Afternoon: Calories / Points **B**

Evening: Calories / Points **C**

DATE: / /   Bed ▢ : ▢   Awake ▢ : ▢   Hours ▢

NOTES

TO DO

Today I am grateful for:

MEAL PLANNER - Tomorrows Meals Organised!

TODAYS HEALTHY HABITS - Five a day - Colour me in - Water - Fruit & Veggies

ACTIVITY

Total Steps

Total Floors / Flights

EXERCISE

Completed Exercise Routine

3 x 1 Min / Exercise 1

3 x 1 Min / Exercise 2

3 x 1 Min / Exercise 3

Calorie / Points Total

(A) + (B) + (C)

Beverage Total

Weight Loss Calorie Goal

Amount of Calories Required to Lose Weight Today...

Maintenance Goal

Amount of Calories Required to Maintain Weight Today...

BREAKFAST / MORNING

Calories / Points ✓

LUNCH / AFTERNOON

DINNER / EVENING

Morning: Calories / Points **A**

Afternoon: Calories / Points **B**

Evening: Calories / Points **C**

DATE: / / Bed : Awake : Hours

NOTES

Today I am grateful for:

TO DO

MEAL PLANNER - Tomorrows Meals Organised!

TODAYS HEALTHY HABITS - Five a day - Colour me in - Water - Fruit & Veggies

ACTIVITY

Total Steps

Total Floors / Flights

EXERCISE

Completed Exercise Routine

3 x 1 Min / Exercise 1

3 x 1 Min / Exercise 2

3 x 1 Min / Exercise 3

Calorie / Points Total

(A) + (B) + (C)

Beverage Total

Weight Loss Calorie Goal

Amount of Calories Required to Lose Weight Today...

Maintenance Goal

Amount of Calories Required to Maintain Weight Today...

BREAKFAST / MORNING

Calories / Points

LUNCH / AFTERNOON

DINNER / EVENING

Morning: Calories / Points   Afternoon: Calories / Points   Evening: Calories / Points

A   **B**   **C**

DATE: /   /   Bed   [:]   Awake   [:]   Hours [   ]

NOTES   TO DO

- [ ]
- [ ]
- [ ]
- [ ]
- [ ]

Today I am grateful for:

MEAL PLANNER - Tomorrows Meals Organised!

TODAYS HEALTHY HABITS - Five a day - Colour me in - Water - Fruit & Veggies

ACTIVITY

Total Steps [   ]

Total Floors / Flights [   ]

EXERCISE

Completed Exercise Routine

3 x 1 Min / Exercise 1   [ ] [ ] [ ]

3 x 1 Min / Exercise 2   [ ] [ ] [ ]

3 x 1 Min / Exercise 3   [ ] [ ] [ ]

Calorie / Points Total

[   ]   (A) + (B) + (C) ←

Beverage Total

[   ] ✓ ←

Weight Loss Calorie Goal

[   ]   *Amount of Calories Required to Lose Weight Today...*

Maintenance Goal

[   ]   *Amount of Calories Required to Maintain Weight Today...*

BREAKFAST / MORNING

Calories / Points ✓

LUNCH / AFTERNOON

DINNER / EVENING

Morning: Calories / Points
A

Afternoon: Calories / Points
B

Evening: Calories / Points
C

DATE: /   /   Bed   :   Awake   :   Hours

NOTES
TO DO

Today I am grateful for:

MEAL PLANNER - Tomorrows Meals Organised!

TODAYS HEALTHY HABITS - Five a day - Colour me in - Water - Fruit & Veggies

ACTIVITY

Total Steps

Total Floors / Flights

Calorie / Points Total

(A) + (B) + (C)

Beverage Total

EXERCISE

Completed Exercise Routine

3 x 1 Min / Exercise 1

3 x 1 Min / Exercise 2

3 x 1 Min / Exercise 3

Weight Loss Calorie Goal

Amount of Calories Required to Lose Weight Today...

Maintenance Goal

Amount of Calories Required to Maintain Weight Today...

BREAKFAST / MORNING

Calories / Points

LUNCH / AFTERNOON

DINNER / EVENING

Morning: Calories / Points **A**

Afternoon: Calories / Points **B**

Evening: Calories / Points **C**

DATE: / /   Bed [:]   Awake [:]   Hours [ ]

NOTES

TO DO

Today I am grateful for:

MEAL PLANNER - Tomorrows Meals Organised!

TODAYS HEALTHY HABITS - Five a day - Colour me in - Water - Fruit & Veggies

ACTIVITY

Total Steps [ ]

Total Floors / Flights [ ]

EXERCISE

Completed Exercise Routine

3 x 1 Min / Exercise 1

3 x 1 Min / Exercise 2

3 x 1 Min / Exercise 3

Calorie / Points Total

[ ]   (A) + (B) + (C) ←

Beverage Total

[ ]

Weight Loss Calorie Goal

[ ]   *Amount of Calories Required to Lose Weight Today...*

Maintenance Goal

[ ]   *Amount of Calories Required to Maintain Weight Today...*

BREAKFAST / MORNING

Calories / Points ✓

LUNCH / AFTERNOON

DINNER / EVENING

Morning: Calories / Points **A**

Afternoon: Calories / Points **B**

Evening: Calories / Points **C**

DATE: /   /   Bed :   Awake :   Hours

NOTES

TO DO

Today I am grateful for:

MEAL PLANNER - Tomorrows Meals Organised!

TODAYS HEALTHY HABITS - Five a day - Colour me in - Water - Fruit & Veggies

ACTIVITY

Total Steps

Total Floors / Flights

Calorie / Points Total

(A) + (B) + (C)

Beverage Total

EXERCISE

Completed Exercise Routine

3 x 1 Min / Exercise 1

3 x 1 Min / Exercise 2

3 x 1 Min / Exercise 3

Weight Loss Calorie Goal

Amount of Calories Required to Lose Weight Today...

Maintenance Goal

Amount of Calories Required to Maintain Weight Today...

BREAKFAST / MORNING

Calories / Points

LUNCH / AFTERNOON

DINNER / EVENING

Morning: Calories / Points **A**

Afternoon: Calories / Points **B**

Evening: Calories / Points **C**

DATE: / / Bed : Awake : Hours

NOTES

TO DO

Today I am grateful for:

MEAL PLANNER - Tomorrows Meals Organised!

TODAYS HEALTHY HABITS - Five a day - Colour me in - Water - Fruit & Veggies

ACTIVITY

Total Steps

Total Floors / Flights

EXERCISE

Completed Exercise Routine

3 x 1 Min / Exercise 1

3 x 1 Min / Exercise 2

3 x 1 Min / Exercise 3

Calorie / Points Total

(A) + (B) + (C)

Beverage Total

Weight Loss Calorie Goal

Amount of Calories Required to Lose Weight Today...

Maintenance Goal

Amount of Calories Required to Maintain Weight Today...

BREAKFAST / MORNING

Calories / Points

LUNCH / AFTERNOON

DINNER / EVENING

Morning: Calories / Points **A**

Afternoon: Calories / Points **B**

Evening: Calories / Points **C**

DATE: ___ / ___ / ___   Bed ☐ : ☐   Awake ☐ : ☐   Hours ☐

NOTES

TO DO
☐
☐
☐
☐
☐

Today I am grateful for:

MEAL PLANNER - Tomorrows Meals Organised!

TODAYS HEALTHY HABITS - Five a day - Colour me in - Water - Fruit & Veggies

ACTIVITY

Total Steps ☐

Total Floors / Flights ☐

EXERCISE

Completed Exercise Routine

3 x 1 Min / Exercise 1 ☐ ☐ ☐

3 x 1 Min / Exercise 2 ☐ ☐ ☐

3 x 1 Min / Exercise 3 ☐ ☐ ☐

Calorie / Points Total

☐ (A) + (B) + (C) ←

Beverage Total

☐ ✓ ←

Weight Loss Calorie Goal

☐   *Amount of Calories Required to Lose Weight Today...*

Maintenance Goal

☐   *Amount of Calories Required to Maintain Weight Today...*

BREAKFAST / MORNING

Calories / Points ✓

LUNCH / AFTERNOON

✓

DINNER / EVENING

✓

Morning: Calories / Points
Afternoon: Calories / Points
Evening: Calories / Points

A **B** **C**

DATE: /   /   Bed :   Awake :   Hours

NOTES   TO DO

Today I am grateful for:

MEAL PLANNER - Tomorrows Meals Organised!

TODAYS HEALTHY HABITS - Five a day - Colour me in - Water - Fruit & Veggies

ACTIVITY

Total Steps

Total Floors / Flights

Calorie / Points Total

(A) + (B) + (C)

Beverage Total

EXERCISE

Completed Exercise Routine

3 x 1 Min / Exercise 1

3 x 1 Min / Exercise 2

3 x 1 Min / Exercise 3

Weight Loss Calorie Goal

Amount of Calories Required to Lose Weight Today...

Maintenance Goal

Amount of Calories Required to Maintain Weight Today...

BREAKFAST / MORNING

Calories / Points

LUNCH / AFTERNOON

DINNER / EVENING

Morning: Calories / Points **A**

Afternoon: Calories / Points **B**

Evening: Calories / Points **C**

DATE: / /   Bed : Awake :   Hours

NOTES

TO DO

Today I am grateful for:

MEAL PLANNER - Tomorrows Meals Organised!

TODAYS HEALTHY HABITS - Five a day - Colour me in - Water - Fruit & Veggies

ACTIVITY

Total Steps

Total Floors / Flights

EXERCISE

Completed Exercise Routine

3 x 1 Min / Exercise 1

3 x 1 Min / Exercise 2

3 x 1 Min / Exercise 3

Calorie / Points Total

(A) + (B) + (C)

Beverage Total

Weight Loss Calorie Goal

Amount of Calories Required to Lose Weight Today...

Maintenance Goal

Amount of Calories Required to Maintain Weight Today...

BREAKFAST / MORNING

Calories / Points

LUNCH / AFTERNOON

DINNER / EVENING

Morning: Calories / Points **A**

Afternoon: Calories / Points **B**

Evening: Calories / Points **C**

DATE: /   /   Bed [:]   Awake [:]   Hours [   ]

NOTES

TO DO

Today I am grateful for:

MEAL PLANNER - Tomorrows Meals Organised!

TODAYS HEALTHY HABITS - Five a day - Colour me in - Water - Fruit & Veggies

ACTIVITY

Total Steps

Total Floors / Flights

Calorie / Points Total

(A) + (B) + (C)

Beverage Total

EXERCISE

Completed Exercise Routine

3 x 1 Min / Exercise 1

3 x 1 Min / Exercise 2

3 x 1 Min / Exercise 3

Weight Loss Calorie Goal

Amount of Calories Required to Lose Weight Today...

Maintenance Goal

Amount of Calories Required to Maintain Weight Today...

BREAKFAST / MORNING

Calories / Points ✓

LUNCH / AFTERNOON

DINNER / EVENING

Morning: Calories / Points   Afternoon: Calories / Points   Evening: Calories / Points

A   **B**   **C**

DATE: /   /   Bed [:]   Awake [:]   Hours [   ]

NOTES

TO DO

Today I am grateful for:

MEAL PLANNER - Tomorrows Meals Organised!

TODAYS HEALTHY HABITS - Five a day - Colour me in - Water - Fruit & Veggies

ACTIVITY

Total Steps [   ]

Total Floors / Flights [   ]

EXERCISE

Completed Exercise Routine

3 x 1 Min / Exercise 1

3 x 1 Min / Exercise 2

3 x 1 Min / Exercise 3

Calorie / Points Total

[   ]   (A) + (B) + (C) ←

Beverage Total

[   ] ✓

Weight Loss Calorie Goal

[   ]   *Amount of Calories Required to Lose Weight Today...*

Maintenance Goal

[   ]   *Amount of Calories Required to Maintain Weight Today...*

BREAKFAST / MORNING

Calories / Points

LUNCH / AFTERNOON

DINNER / EVENING

Morning: Calories / Points **A**

Afternoon: Calories / Points **B**

Evening: Calories / Points **C**

DATE: /   /   Bed   :   Awake   :   Hours

NOTES

TO DO

Today I am grateful for:

MEAL PLANNER - Tomorrows Meals Organised!

TODAYS HEALTHY HABITS - Five a day - Colour me in - Water - Fruit & Veggies

ACTIVITY

Total Steps

Total Floors / Flights

Calorie / Points Total

(A) + (B) + (C)

Beverage Total

EXERCISE

Completed Exercise Routine

3 x 1 Min / Exercise 1

3 x 1 Min / Exercise 2

3 x 1 Min / Exercise 3

Weight Loss Calorie Goal

Amount of Calories Required to Lose Weight Today...

Maintenance Goal

Amount of Calories Required to Maintain Weight Today...

BREAKFAST / MORNING

Calories / Points ✓

LUNCH / AFTERNOON

✓

DINNER / EVENING

✓

Morning: Calories / Points **A**

Afternoon: Calories / Points **B**

Evening: Calories / Points **C**

DATE: / /   **Bed** : **Awake** : **Hours**

NOTES

TO DO

Today I am grateful for:

MEAL PLANNER - Tomorrows Meals Organised!

TODAYS HEALTHY HABITS - Five a day - Colour me in - Water - Fruit & Veggies

ACTIVITY

Total Steps

Total Floors / Flights

EXERCISE

Completed Exercise Routine

3 x 1 Min / Exercise 1

3 x 1 Min / Exercise 2

3 x 1 Min / Exercise 3

Calorie / Points Total

(A) + (B) + (C)

Beverage Total

Weight Loss Calorie Goal

Amount of Calories Required to Lose Weight Today...

Maintenance Goal

Amount of Calories Required to Maintain Weight Today...

BREAKFAST / MORNING

Calories / Points

LUNCH / AFTERNOON

DINNER / EVENING

Morning: Calories / Points
Afternoon: Calories / Points
Evening: Calories / Points

A **B** **C**

DATE: /   /   Bed [:]   Awake [:]   Hours [   ]

NOTES

TO DO

Today I am grateful for:

MEAL PLANNER - Tomorrows Meals Organised!

TODAYS HEALTHY HABITS - Five a day - Colour me in - Water - Fruit & Veggies

ACTIVITY

Total Steps

Total Floors / Flights

EXERCISE

Completed Exercise Routine

3 x 1 Min / Exercise 1

3 x 1 Min / Exercise 2

3 x 1 Min / Exercise 3

Calorie / Points Total

(A) + (B) + (C) ←

Beverage Total

Weight Loss Calorie Goal

Amount of Calories Required to Lose Weight Today...

Maintenance Goal

Amount of Calories Required to Maintain Weight Today...

BREAKFAST / MORNING

Calories / Points ✓

LUNCH / AFTERNOON

DINNER / EVENING

Morning: Calories / Points
A

Afternoon: Calories / Points
B

Evening: Calories / Points
C

DATE: /   /   Bed   :   Awake   :   Hours

NOTES

Today I am grateful for:

TO DO

MEAL PLANNER - Tomorrows Meals Organised!

TODAYS HEALTHY HABITS - Five a day - Colour me in - Water - Fruit & Veggies

ACTIVITY

Total Steps

Total Floors / Flights

EXERCISE

Completed Exercise Routine

3 x 1 Min / Exercise 1

3 x 1 Min / Exercise 2

3 x 1 Min / Exercise 3

Calorie / Points Total

(A) + (B) + (C)

Beverage Total

Weight Loss Calorie Goal

Amount of Calories Required to Lose Weight Today...

Maintenance Goal

Amount of Calories Required to Maintain Weight Today...

BREAKFAST / MORNING

Calories / Points ✓

LUNCH / AFTERNOON

DINNER / EVENING

Morning: Calories / Points
A

Afternoon: Calories / Points
B

Evening: Calories / Points
C

DATE: ___/___/___   Bed ☐:☐   Awake ☐:☐   Hours ☐

NOTES

Today I am grateful for:

TO DO

☐
☐
☐
☐
☐

MEAL PLANNER - Tomorrows Meals Organised!

TODAYS HEALTHY HABITS - Five a day - Colour me in - Water - Fruit & Veggies

ACTIVITY

Total Steps ☐
Total Floors / Flights ☐

EXERCISE

Completed Exercise Routine

3 x 1 Min / Exercise 1   ☐ ☐ ☐
3 x 1 Min / Exercise 2   ☐ ☐ ☐
3 x 1 Min / Exercise 3   ☐ ☐ ☐

Calorie / Points Total

☐   (A) + (B) + (C) ←

Beverage Total

☐   ✓

Weight Loss Calorie Goal

☐   *Amount of Calories Required to Lose Weight Today...*

Maintenance Goal

☐   *Amount of Calories Required to Maintain Weight Today...*

BREAKFAST / MORNING

Calories / Points ✓

LUNCH / AFTERNOON

DINNER / EVENING

Morning: Calories / Points **A**

Afternoon: Calories / Points **B**

Evening: Calories / Points **C**

DATE: / /   Bed : Awake : Hours

NOTES

TO DO

☐
☐
☐
☐
☐

Today I am grateful for:

MEAL PLANNER - Tomorrows Meals Organised!

TODAYS HEALTHY HABITS - Five a day - Colour me in - Water - Fruit & Veggies

ACTIVITY

Total Steps

Total Floors / Flights

Calorie / Points Total

(A) + (B) + (C)

Beverage Total

EXERCISE

Completed Exercise Routine

3 x 1 Min / Exercise 1

3 x 1 Min / Exercise 2

3 x 1 Min / Exercise 3

Weight Loss Calorie Goal

Amount of Calories Required to Lose Weight Today...

Maintenance Goal

Amount of Calories Required to Maintain Weight Today...

BREAKFAST / MORNING   Calories / Points ✓

LUNCH / AFTERNOON   ✓

DINNER / EVENING   ✓

Morning: Calories / Points   Afternoon: Calories / Points   Evening: Calories / Points

A   **B**   **C**

DATE: /   /   Bed :   Awake :   Hours

NOTES

TO DO

Today I am grateful for:

MEAL PLANNER - Tomorrows Meals Organised!

TODAYS HEALTHY HABITS - Five a day - Colour me in - Water - Fruit & Veggies

ACTIVITY

Total Steps

Total Floors / Flights

EXERCISE

Completed Exercise Routine

3 x 1 Min / Exercise 1

3 x 1 Min / Exercise 2

3 x 1 Min / Exercise 3

Calorie / Points Total

(A) + (B) + (C)

Beverage Total

Weight Loss Calorie Goal

Amount of Calories Required to Lose Weight Today...

Maintenance Goal

Amount of Calories Required to Maintain Weight Today...

BREAKFAST / MORNING

Calories / Points

LUNCH / AFTERNOON

DINNER / EVENING

Morning: Calories / Points **A**

Afternoon: Calories / Points **B**

Evening: Calories / Points **C**

DATE: /   /   Bed [:]   Awake [:]   Hours [   ]

NOTES

TO DO

Today I am grateful for:

MEAL PLANNER - Tomorrows Meals Organised!

TODAYS HEALTHY HABITS - Five a day - Colour me in - Water - Fruit & Veggies

ACTIVITY

Total Steps [   ]

Total Floors / Flights [   ]

EXERCISE

Completed Exercise Routine

3 x 1 Min / Exercise 1

3 x 1 Min / Exercise 2

3 x 1 Min / Exercise 3

Calorie / Points Total

[   ]   (A) + (B) + (C) ←

Beverage Total

[   ]

Weight Loss Calorie Goal

[   ]   *Amount of Calories Required to Lose Weight Today...*

Maintenance Goal

[   ]   *Amount of Calories Required to Maintain Weight Today...*

BREAKFAST / MORNING

Calories / Points ✓

LUNCH / AFTERNOON

✓

DINNER / EVENING

✓

Morning: Calories / Points

A

Afternoon: Calories / Points

B

Evening: Calories / Points

C

DATE: /   /   Bed :   Awake :   Hours

NOTES

TO DO

Today I am grateful for:

MEAL PLANNER - Tomorrows Meals Organised!

TODAYS HEALTHY HABITS - Five a day - Colour me in - Water - Fruit & Veggies

ACTIVITY

Total Steps

Total Floors / Flights

Calorie / Points Total

(A) + (B) + (C)

Beverage Total

EXERCISE

Completed Exercise Routine

3 x 1 Min / Exercise 1

3 x 1 Min / Exercise 2

3 x 1 Min / Exercise 3

Weight Loss Calorie Goal

Amount of Calories Required to Lose Weight Today...

Maintenance Goal

Amount of Calories Required to Maintain Weight Today...

BREAKFAST / MORNING

Calories / Points

LUNCH / AFTERNOON

DINNER / EVENING

Morning: Calories / Points **A**

Afternoon: Calories / Points **B**

Evening: Calories / Points **C**

DATE: /   /   Bed   :   Awake   :   Hours

NOTES

TO DO

Today I am grateful for:

MEAL PLANNER - Tomorrows Meals Organised!

TODAYS HEALTHY HABITS - Five a day - Colour me in - Water - Fruit & Veggies

ACTIVITY

Total Steps

Total Floors / Flights

EXERCISE

Completed Exercise Routine

3 x 1 Min / Exercise 1

3 x 1 Min / Exercise 2

3 x 1 Min / Exercise 3

Calorie / Points Total

(A) + (B) + (C)

Beverage Total

Weight Loss Calorie Goal

Amount of Calories Required to Lose Weight Today...

Maintenance Goal

Amount of Calories Required to Maintain Weight Today...

BREAKFAST / MORNING

Calories / Points

LUNCH / AFTERNOON

DINNER / EVENING

Morning: Calories / Points

A

Afternoon: Calories / Points

B

Evening: Calories / Points

C

DATE: /   /   Bed :   Awake :   Hours

NOTES
TO DO

Today I am grateful for:

MEAL PLANNER - Tomorrows Meals Organised!

TODAYS HEALTHY HABITS - Five a day - Colour me in - Water - Fruit & Veggies

ACTIVITY

Total Steps

Total Floors / Flights

Calorie / Points Total

(A) + (B) + (C)

Beverage Total

EXERCISE

Completed Exercise Routine

3 x 1 Min / Exercise 1

3 x 1 Min / Exercise 2

3 x 1 Min / Exercise 3

Weight Loss Calorie Goal

Amount of Calories Required to Lose Weight Today...

Maintenance Goal

Amount of Calories Required to Maintain Weight Today...

BREAKFAST / MORNING

Calories / Points ✓

LUNCH / AFTERNOON

DINNER / EVENING

Morning: Calories / Points
A

Afternoon: Calories / Points
B

Evening: Calories / Points
C

DATE: /   /   Bed   :   Awake   :   Hours

NOTES

TO DO

Today I am grateful for:

MEAL PLANNER - Tomorrows Meals Organised!

TODAYS HEALTHY HABITS - Five a day - Colour me in - Water - Fruit & Veggies

ACTIVITY

Total Steps

Total Floors / Flights

Calorie / Points Total

(A) + (B) + (C)

Beverage Total

EXERCISE

Completed Exercise Routine

3 x 1 Min / Exercise 1

3 x 1 Min / Exercise 2

3 x 1 Min / Exercise 3

Weight Loss Calorie Goal

Amount of Calories Required to Lose Weight Today...

Maintenance Goal

Amount of Calories Required to Maintain Weight Today...

BREAKFAST / MORNING

Calories / Points

LUNCH / AFTERNOON

DINNER / EVENING

Morning: Calories / Points **A**

Afternoon: Calories / Points **B**

Evening: Calories / Points **C**

DATE: /   /   Bed   :   Awake   :   Hours

NOTES

TO DO

Today I am grateful for:

MEAL PLANNER - Tomorrows Meals Organised!

TODAYS HEALTHY HABITS - Five a day - Colour me in - Water - Fruit & Veggies

ACTIVITY

Total Steps

Total Floors / Flights

Calorie / Points Total

(A) + (B) + (C)

Beverage Total

EXERCISE

Completed Exercise Routine

3 x 1 Min / Exercise 1

3 x 1 Min / Exercise 2

3 x 1 Min / Exercise 3

Weight Loss Calorie Goal

Amount of Calories Required to Lose Weight Today...

Maintenance Goal

Amount of Calories Required to Maintain Weight Today...

BREAKFAST / MORNING

Calories / Points ✓

LUNCH / AFTERNOON

DINNER / EVENING

Morning: Calories / Points   Afternoon: Calories / Points   Evening: Calories / Points

A   **B**   **C**

DATE: / /   Bed ☐ : ☐   Awake ☐ : ☐   Hours ☐

NOTES

TO DO
☐
☐
☐
☐
☐

Today I am grateful for:

MEAL PLANNER - Tomorrows Meals Organised!

TODAYS HEALTHY HABITS - Five a day - Colour me in - Water - Fruit & Veggies

ACTIVITY

Total Steps ☐

Total Floors / Flights ☐

EXERCISE

Completed Exercise Routine

3 x 1 Min / Exercise 1 ☐ ☐ ☐

3 x 1 Min / Exercise 2 ☐ ☐ ☐

3 x 1 Min / Exercise 3 ☐ ☐ ☐

Calorie / Points Total

☐   (A) + (B) + (C) ←

Beverage Total

☐ ←

Weight Loss Calorie Goal

☐   *Amount of Calories Required to Lose Weight Today...*

Maintenance Goal

☐   *Amount of Calories Required to Maintain Weight Today...*

BREAKFAST / MORNING

Calories / Points ✓

LUNCH / AFTERNOON

✓

DINNER / EVENING

✓

Morning: Calories / Points **A**

Afternoon: Calories / Points **B**

Evening: Calories / Points **C**

DATE: /   /   Bed   :   Awake   :   Hours

NOTES

TO DO

Today I am grateful for:

MEAL PLANNER - Tomorrows Meals Organised!

TODAYS HEALTHY HABITS - Five a day - Colour me in - Water - Fruit & Veggies

ACTIVITY

Total Steps

Total Floors / Flights

Calorie / Points Total

(A) + (B) + (C)

Beverage Total

EXERCISE

Completed Exercise Routine

3 x 1 Min / Exercise 1

3 x 1 Min / Exercise 2

3 x 1 Min / Exercise 3

Weight Loss Calorie Goal

Amount of Calories Required to Lose Weight Today...

Maintenance Goal

Amount of Calories Required to Maintain Weight Today...

BREAKFAST / MORNING

Calories / Points ✓

LUNCH / AFTERNOON

Calories / Points ✓

DINNER / EVENING

Calories / Points ✓

Morning: Calories / Points
A

Afternoon: Calories / Points
B

Evening: Calories / Points
C

DATE: _/_/_ **Bed** ☐:☐ **Awake** ☐:☐ **Hours** ☐

NOTES

TO DO
- ☐
- ☐
- ☐
- ☐
- ☐

Today I am grateful for:

MEAL PLANNER - Tomorrows Meals Organised!

TODAYS HEALTHY HABITS - Five a day - Colour me in - Water - Fruit & Veggies

ACTIVITY

Total Steps: ☐

Total Floors / Flights: ☐

EXERCISE

Completed Exercise Routine

3 x 1 Min / Exercise 1 ☐ ☐ ☐

3 x 1 Min / Exercise 2 ☐ ☐ ☐

3 x 1 Min / Exercise 3 ☐ ☐ ☐

Calorie / Points Total

☐ (A) + (B) + (C) ←

Beverage Total

☐ ✓

Weight Loss Calorie Goal

☐ *Amount of Calories Required to Lose Weight Today...*

Maintenance Goal

☐ *Amount of Calories Required to Maintain Weight Today...*

BREAKFAST / MORNING

Calories / Points

LUNCH / AFTERNOON

Calories / Points

DINNER / EVENING

Calories / Points

Morning: Calories / Points **A**

Afternoon: Calories / Points **B**

Evening: Calories / Points **C**

DATE: / /   Bed : Awake : Hours

NOTES

TO DO

Today I am grateful for:

MEAL PLANNER - Tomorrows Meals Organised!

TODAYS HEALTHY HABITS - Five a day - Colour me in - Water - Fruit & Veggies

ACTIVITY

Total Steps

Total Floors / Flights

EXERCISE

Completed Exercise Routine

3 x 1 Min / Exercise 1

3 x 1 Min / Exercise 2

3 x 1 Min / Exercise 3

Calorie / Points Total

(A) + (B) + (C)

Beverage Total

Weight Loss Calorie Goal

Amount of Calories Required to Lose Weight Today...

Maintenance Goal

Amount of Calories Required to Maintain Weight Today...

BREAKFAST / MORNING

Calories / Points

LUNCH / AFTERNOON

Calories / Points

DINNER / EVENING

Morning: Calories / Points **A**

Afternoon: Calories / Points **B**

Evening: Calories / Points **C**

DATE: /   /   Bed :   Awake :   Hours

NOTES   TO DO

Today I am grateful for:

MEAL PLANNER - Tomorrows Meals Organised!

TODAYS HEALTHY HABITS - Five a day - Colour me in - Water - Fruit & Veggies

ACTIVITY

Total Steps

Total Floors / Flights

Calorie / Points Total

(A) + (B) + (C)

Beverage Total

EXERCISE

Completed Exercise Routine

3 x 1 Min / Exercise 1

3 x 1 Min / Exercise 2

3 x 1 Min / Exercise 3

Weight Loss Calorie Goal

Amount of Calories Required to Lose Weight Today...

Maintenance Goal

Amount of Calories Required to Maintain Weight Today...

BREAKFAST / MORNING

Calories / Points

LUNCH / AFTERNOON

DINNER / EVENING

Morning: Calories / Points **A**

Afternoon: Calories / Points **B**

Evening: Calories / Points **C**

DATE: / /   Bed :   Awake :   Hours

NOTES

Today I am grateful for:

TO DO

MEAL PLANNER - Tomorrows Meals Organised!

TODAYS HEALTHY HABITS - Five a day - Colour me in - Water - Fruit & Veggies

ACTIVITY

Total Steps

Total Floors / Flights

EXERCISE

Completed Exercise Routine

3 x 1 Min / Exercise 1

3 x 1 Min / Exercise 2

3 x 1 Min / Exercise 3

Calorie / Points Total

(A) + (B) + (C)

Beverage Total

Weight Loss Calorie Goal

Amount of Calories Required to Lose Weight Today...

Maintenance Goal

Amount of Calories Required to Maintain Weight Today...

BREAKFAST / MORNING

Calories / Points

LUNCH / AFTERNOON

DINNER / EVENING

Morning: Calories / Points **A**

Afternoon: Calories / Points **B**

Evening: Calories / Points **C**

DATE: /   /   Bed :   Awake :   Hours

NOTES

TO DO

Today I am grateful for:

MEAL PLANNER - Tomorrows Meals Organised!

TODAYS HEALTHY HABITS - Five a day - Colour me in - Water - Fruit & Veggies

ACTIVITY

Total Steps

Total Floors / Flights

EXERCISE

Completed Exercise Routine

3 x 1 Min / Exercise 1

3 x 1 Min / Exercise 2

3 x 1 Min / Exercise 3

Calorie / Points Total

(A) + (B) + (C)

Beverage Total

Weight Loss Calorie Goal

Amount of Calories Required to Lose Weight Today...

Maintenance Goal

Amount of Calories Required to Maintain Weight Today...

BREAKFAST / MORNING

Calories / Points

LUNCH / AFTERNOON

DINNER / EVENING

Morning: Calories / Points   Afternoon: Calories / Points   Evening: Calories / Points

A **B** **C**

DATE: /   /   Bed [:]   Awake [:]   Hours [ ]

NOTES

TO DO

Today I am grateful for:

MEAL PLANNER - Tomorrows Meals Organised!

TODAYS HEALTHY HABITS - Five a day - Colour me in - Water - Fruit & Veggies

ACTIVITY

Total Steps [ ]

Total Floors / Flights [ ]

EXERCISE

Completed Exercise Routine

3 x 1 Min / Exercise 1

3 x 1 Min / Exercise 2

3 x 1 Min / Exercise 3

Calorie / Points Total

[ ]   (A) + (B) + (C) ←

Beverage Total

[ ]

Weight Loss Calorie Goal

[ ]   *Amount of Calories Required to Lose Weight Today...*

Maintenance Goal

[ ]   *Amount of Calories Required to Maintain Weight Today...*

BREAKFAST / MORNING

Calories / Points

LUNCH / AFTERNOON

DINNER / EVENING

Morning: Calories / Points   **A**
Afternoon: Calories / Points   **B**
Evening: Calories / Points   **C**

DATE: /   /   Bed [:]   Awake [:]   Hours [   ]

NOTES

TO DO

Today I am grateful for:

MEAL PLANNER - Tomorrows Meals Organised!

TODAYS HEALTHY HABITS - Five a day - Colour me in - Water - Fruit & Veggies

ACTIVITY

Total Steps [   ]

Total Floors / Flights [   ]

EXERCISE

Completed Exercise Routine

3 x 1 Min / Exercise 1 ☐ ☐ ☐

3 x 1 Min / Exercise 2 ☐ ☐ ☐

3 x 1 Min / Exercise 3 ☐ ☐ ☐

Calorie / Points Total

[   ] (A) + (B) + (C) ◄

Beverage Total

[   ] ☑ ◄

Weight Loss Calorie Goal

[   ] *Amount of Calories Required to Lose Weight Today...*

Maintenance Goal

[   ] *Amount of Calories Required to Maintain Weight Today...*

BREAKFAST / MORNING

Calories / Points

LUNCH / AFTERNOON

DINNER / EVENING

Morning: Calories / Points **A**

Afternoon: Calories / Points **B**

Evening: Calories / Points **C**

DATE: /   /   Bed   :   Awake   :   Hours

NOTES

TO DO

Today I am grateful for:

MEAL PLANNER - Tomorrows Meals Organised!

TODAYS HEALTHY HABITS - Five a day - Colour me in - Water - Fruit & Veggies

ACTIVITY

Total Steps

Total Floors / Flights

Calorie / Points Total

(A) + (B) + (C)

Beverage Total

EXERCISE

Completed Exercise Routine

3 x 1 Min / Exercise 1

3 x 1 Min / Exercise 2

3 x 1 Min / Exercise 3

Weight Loss Calorie Goal

Amount of Calories Required to Lose Weight Today...

Maintenance Goal

Amount of Calories Required to Maintain Weight Today...

BREAKFAST / MORNING

Calories / Points ✓

LUNCH / AFTERNOON

DINNER / EVENING

Morning: Calories / Points **A**

Afternoon: Calories / Points **B**

Evening: Calories / Points **C**

DATE: /   /   Bed [:]   Awake [:]   Hours [   ]

NOTES   TO DO

☐
☐
☐
☐
Today I am grateful for: ☐

MEAL PLANNER - Tomorrows Meals Organised!

TODAYS HEALTHY HABITS - Five a day - Colour me in - Water - Fruit & Veggies

ACTIVITY

Total Steps [   ]

Total Floors / Flights [   ]

EXERCISE

Completed Exercise Routine

3 x 1 Min / Exercise 1

3 x 1 Min / Exercise 2

3 x 1 Min / Exercise 3

Calorie / Points Total

[   ]   (A) + (B) + (C)

Beverage Total

[   ] ✓

Weight Loss Calorie Goal

[   ]   *Amount of Calories Required to Lose Weight Today...*

Maintenance Goal

[   ]   *Amount of Calories Required to Maintain Weight Today...*

BREAKFAST / MORNING | Calories / Points ✓

LUNCH / AFTERNOON ✓

DINNER / EVENING ✓

Morning: Calories / Points **A**

Afternoon: Calories / Points **B**

Evening: Calories / Points **C**

DATE: /   /   Bed :   Awake :   Hours

NOTES

TO DO

Today I am grateful for:

MEAL PLANNER - Tomorrows Meals Organised!

TODAYS HEALTHY HABITS - Five a day - Colour me in - Water - Fruit & Veggies

ACTIVITY

Total Steps

Total Floors / Flights

Calorie / Points Total

(A) + (B) + (C)

Beverage Total

EXERCISE

Completed Exercise Routine

3 x 1 Min / Exercise 1

3 x 1 Min / Exercise 2

3 x 1 Min / Exercise 3

Weight Loss Calorie Goal

Amount of Calories Required to Lose Weight Today...

Maintenance Goal

Amount of Calories Required to Maintain Weight Today...

BREAKFAST / MORNING　　　　　　　　　　　　　　　　　　Calories / Points ✓

LUNCH / AFTERNOON ✓

DINNER / EVENING ✓

Morning: Calories / Points　　Afternoon: Calories / Points　　Evening: Calories / Points

A　　　　**B**　　　　**C**

DATE: ___ / ___ / ___ Bed ___ : ___ Awake ___ : ___ Hours ___

NOTES

TO DO

☐
☐
☐
☐
☐

Today I am grateful for:

MEAL PLANNER - Tomorrows Meals Organised!

TODAYS HEALTHY HABITS - Five a day - Colour me in - Water - Fruit & Veggies

ACTIVITY

Total Steps ___

Total Floors / Flights ___

EXERCISE

Completed Exercise Routine

3 x 1 Min / Exercise 1 ☐ ☐ ☐

3 x 1 Min / Exercise 2 ☐ ☐ ☐

3 x 1 Min / Exercise 3 ☐ ☐ ☐

Calorie / Points Total ___ (A) + (B) + (C) ←

Beverage Total ___ ✓

Weight Loss Calorie Goal ___
Amount of Calories Required to Lose Weight Today...

Maintenance Goal ___
Amount of Calories Required to Maintain Weight Today...

BREAKFAST / MORNING

Calories / Points

LUNCH / AFTERNOON

DINNER / EVENING

Morning: Calories / Points **A**

Afternoon: Calories / Points **B**

Evening: Calories / Points **C**

DATE: / / Bed : Awake : Hours

NOTES

TO DO

Today I am grateful for:

MEAL PLANNER - Tomorrows Meals Organised!

TODAYS HEALTHY HABITS - Five a day - Colour me in - Water - Fruit & Veggies

ACTIVITY

Total Steps

Total Floors / Flights

EXERCISE

Completed Exercise Routine

3 x 1 Min / Exercise 1

3 x 1 Min / Exercise 2

3 x 1 Min / Exercise 3

Calorie / Points Total

(A) + (B) + (C)

Beverage Total

Weight Loss Calorie Goal

Amount of Calories Required to Lose Weight Today...

Maintenance Goal

Amount of Calories Required to Maintain Weight Today...

BREAKFAST / MORNING

Calories / Points

LUNCH / AFTERNOON

DINNER / EVENING

Morning: Calories / Points **A**

Afternoon: Calories / Points **B**

Evening: Calories / Points **C**

DATE: /   /   Bed ☐ : ☐   Awake ☐ : ☐   Hours ☐

NOTES

TO DO
☐
☐
☐
☐
☐

Today I am grateful for:

MEAL PLANNER - Tomorrows Meals Organised!

TODAYS HEALTHY HABITS - Five a day - Colour me in - Water - Fruit & Veggies

ACTIVITY

Total Steps ☐

Total Floors / Flights ☐

EXERCISE

Completed Exercise Routine

3 x 1 Min / Exercise 1   ☐ ☐ ☐

3 x 1 Min / Exercise 2   ☐ ☐ ☐

3 x 1 Min / Exercise 3   ☐ ☐ ☐

Calorie / Points Total

☐   (A) + (B) + (C) ◀

Beverage Total

☐   ✓

Weight Loss Calorie Goal

☐   *Amount of Calories Required to Lose Weight Today...*

Maintenance Goal

☐   *Amount of Calories Required to Maintain Weight Today...*

BREAKFAST / MORNING

Calories / Points

LUNCH / AFTERNOON

DINNER / EVENING

Morning: Calories / Points

A

Afternoon: Calories / Points

B

Evening: Calories / Points

C

DATE: /   /   Bed   [:]   Awake [:]   Hours [   ]

NOTES

TO DO

Today I am grateful for:

MEAL PLANNER - Tomorrows Meals Organised!

TODAYS HEALTHY HABITS - Five a day - Colour me in - Water - Fruit & Veggies

ACTIVITY

Total Steps

Total Floors / Flights

EXERCISE

Completed Exercise Routine

3 x 1 Min / Exercise 1

3 x 1 Min / Exercise 2

3 x 1 Min / Exercise 3

Calorie / Points Total

(A) + (B) + (C)

Beverage Total

Weight Loss Calorie Goal

Amount of Calories Required to Lose Weight Today...

Maintenance Goal

Amount of Calories Required to Maintain Weight Today...

BREAKFAST / MORNING

Calories / Points

LUNCH / AFTERNOON

Calories / Points

DINNER / EVENING

Calories / Points

Morning: Calories / Points **A**

Afternoon: Calories / Points **B**

Evening: Calories / Points **C**

DATE: /   /   Bed   :   Awake   :   Hours

NOTES   TO DO

Today I am grateful for:

MEAL PLANNER - Tomorrows Meals Organised!

TODAYS HEALTHY HABITS - Five a day - Colour me in - Water - Fruit & Veggies

ACTIVITY

Total Steps

Total Floors / Flights

Calorie / Points Total

(A) + (B) + (C)

Beverage Total

EXERCISE

Completed Exercise Routine

3 x 1 Min / Exercise 1

3 x 1 Min / Exercise 2

3 x 1 Min / Exercise 3

Weight Loss Calorie Goal

Amount of Calories Required to Lose Weight Today...

Maintenance Goal

Amount of Calories Required to Maintain Weight Today...

BREAKFAST / MORNING

Calories / Points ✓

LUNCH / AFTERNOON

DINNER / EVENING

Morning: Calories / Points
A

Afternoon: Calories / Points
B

Evening: Calories / Points
C

DATE: /   /   Bed [:]   Awake [:]   Hours [   ]

NOTES

Today I am grateful for:

TO DO

☐
☐
☐
☐
☐

MEAL PLANNER - Tomorrows Meals Organised!

TODAYS HEALTHY HABITS - Five a day - Colour me in - Water - Fruit & Veggies

🥛🥛🥛🥛   🍎🍎🍎🍎   🥕🥕🥕🥕🥕

ACTIVITY

Total Steps [   ]

Total Floors / Flights [   ]

EXERCISE

Completed Exercise Routine

3 x 1 Min / Exercise 1   ☐ ☐ ☐

3 x 1 Min / Exercise 2   ☐ ☐ ☐

3 x 1 Min / Exercise 3   ☐ ☐ ☐

Calorie / Points Total

[   ]   (A) + (B) + (C) ←

Beverage Total

[   ] ✓

Weight Loss Calorie Goal

[   ]   *Amount of Calories Required to Lose Weight Today...*

Maintenance Goal

[   ]   *Amount of Calories Required to Maintain Weight Today...*

BREAKFAST / MORNING

Calories / Points

LUNCH / AFTERNOON

DINNER / EVENING

Morning: Calories / Points **A**

Afternoon: Calories / Points **B**

Evening: Calories / Points **C**

DATE: /   /   Bed [:]   Awake [:]   Hours [   ]

NOTES

TO DO
- [ ]
- [ ]
- [ ]
- [ ]
- [ ]

Today I am grateful for:

MEAL PLANNER - Tomorrows Meals Organised!

TODAYS HEALTHY HABITS - Five a day - Colour me in - Water - Fruit & Veggies

🥛🥛🥛🥛   🍎🍎🍎🍎   🥕🥕🥕🥕🥕

ACTIVITY

Total Steps [   ]

Total Floors / Flights [   ]

EXERCISE

Completed Exercise Routine

3 x 1 Min / Exercise 1   [ ] [ ] [ ]

3 x 1 Min / Exercise 2   [ ] [ ] [ ]

3 x 1 Min / Exercise 3   [ ] [ ] [ ]

Calorie / Points Total

[   ]   (A) + (B) + (C) ←

Beverage Total

[   ] ☕✓ ←

Weight Loss Calorie Goal

[   ]   *Amount of Calories Required to Lose Weight Today...*

Maintenance Goal

[   ]   *Amount of Calories Required to Maintain Weight Today...*

BREAKFAST / MORNING

Calories / Points

LUNCH / AFTERNOON

DINNER / EVENING

Morning: Calories / Points   Afternoon: Calories / Points   Evening: Calories / Points

A   **B**   **C**

DATE: /   /   Bed   :   Awake   :   Hours

NOTES

TO DO

Today I am grateful for:

MEAL PLANNER - Tomorrows Meals Organised!

TODAYS HEALTHY HABITS - Five a day - Colour me in - Water - Fruit & Veggies

ACTIVITY

Total Steps

Total Floors / Flights

EXERCISE

Completed Exercise Routine

3 x 1 Min / Exercise 1

3 x 1 Min / Exercise 2

3 x 1 Min / Exercise 3

Calorie / Points Total

(A) + (B) + (C)

Beverage Total

Weight Loss Calorie Goal

Amount of Calories Required to Lose Weight Today...

Maintenance Goal

Amount of Calories Required to Maintain Weight Today...

BREAKFAST / MORNING

Calories / Points ✓

LUNCH / AFTERNOON

DINNER / EVENING

Morning: Calories / Points
A

Afternoon: Calories / Points
B

Evening: Calories / Points
C

DATE: /   /   Bed [:]   Awake [:]   Hours [   ]

NOTES

TO DO

Today I am grateful for:

MEAL PLANNER - Tomorrows Meals Organised!

TODAYS HEALTHY HABITS - Five a day - Colour me in - Water - Fruit & Veggies

ACTIVITY

Total Steps

Total Floors / Flights

EXERCISE

Completed Exercise Routine

3 x 1 Min / Exercise 1

3 x 1 Min / Exercise 2

3 x 1 Min / Exercise 3

Calorie / Points Total

(A) + (B) + (C)

Beverage Total

Weight Loss Calorie Goal

Amount of Calories Required to Lose Weight Today...

Maintenance Goal

Amount of Calories Required to Maintain Weight Today...

BREAKFAST / MORNING

Calories / Points

LUNCH / AFTERNOON

DINNER / EVENING

Morning: Calories / Points **A**

Afternoon: Calories / Points **B**

Evening: Calories / Points **C**

DATE: / /   Bed :   Awake :   Hours

NOTES

Today I am grateful for:

TO DO

MEAL PLANNER - Tomorrows Meals Organised!

TODAYS HEALTHY HABITS - Five a day - Colour me in - Water - Fruit & Veggies

ACTIVITY

Total Steps

Total Floors / Flights

Calorie / Points Total

(A) + (B) + (C)

Beverage Total

EXERCISE

Completed Exercise Routine

3 x 1 Min / Exercise 1

3 x 1 Min / Exercise 2

3 x 1 Min / Exercise 3

Weight Loss Calorie Goal

Amount of Calories Required to Lose Weight Today...

Maintenance Goal

Amount of Calories Required to Maintain Weight Today...

BREAKFAST / MORNING

Calories / Points ✓

LUNCH / AFTERNOON

DINNER / EVENING

Morning: Calories / Points **A**

Afternoon: Calories / Points **B**

Evening: Calories / Points **C**

DATE: /   /   Bed   :   Awake   :   Hours

NOTES

TO DO

Today I am grateful for:

MEAL PLANNER - Tomorrows Meals Organised!

TODAYS HEALTHY HABITS - Five a day - Colour me in - Water - Fruit & Veggies

ACTIVITY

Total Steps

Total Floors / Flights

Calorie / Points Total

(A) + (B) + (C)

Beverage Total

EXERCISE

Completed Exercise Routine

3 x 1 Min / Exercise 1

3 x 1 Min / Exercise 2

3 x 1 Min / Exercise 3

Weight Loss Calorie Goal

Amount of Calories Required to Lose Weight Today...

Maintenance Goal

Amount of Calories Required to Maintain Weight Today...

BREAKFAST / MORNING

Calories / Points ✓

LUNCH / AFTERNOON

✓

DINNER / EVENING

✓

Morning: Calories / Points **A**

Afternoon: Calories / Points **B**

Evening: Calories / Points **C**

DATE: / /   Bed ☐ : ☐   Awake ☐ : ☐   Hours ☐

NOTES

Today I am grateful for:

TO DO

☐
☐
☐
☐
☐

MEAL PLANNER - Tomorrows Meals Organised!

TODAYS HEALTHY HABITS - Five a day - Colour me in - Water - Fruit & Veggies

ACTIVITY

Total Steps ☐

Total Floors / Flights ☐

EXERCISE

Completed Exercise Routine

3 x 1 Min / Exercise 1 ☐ ☐ ☐

3 x 1 Min / Exercise 2 ☐ ☐ ☐

3 x 1 Min / Exercise 3 ☐ ☐ ☐

Calorie / Points Total

☐ (A) + (B) + (C) ←

Beverage Total

☐ ☑

Weight Loss Calorie Goal

☐ *Amount of Calories Required to Lose Weight Today...*

Maintenance Goal

☐ *Amount of Calories Required to Maintain Weight Today...*

BREAKFAST / MORNING

Calories / Points

LUNCH / AFTERNOON

DINNER / EVENING

Morning: Calories / Points **A**

Afternoon: Calories / Points **B**

Evening: Calories / Points **C**

FOOD LIBRARY - BREAKFAST

FOOD ITEM　　　　　CALORIE CALCULATION →　　Calories Per 1 Gram　　Portion, Points, Serving Or Weight　　Total Calories

SET MENUS *FOR* BREAKFAST

Name	Calories

Menu 1 — Calorie Total

Name	Calories

Menu 2 — Calorie Total

Name	Calories

Menu 3 — Calorie Total

Name	Calories

Menu 4 — Calorie Total

Name	Calories

Menu 5 — Calorie Total

Name	Calories

Menu 6 — Calorie Total

FOOD LIBRARY - LUNCH

FOOD ITEM   CALORIE CALCULATION →   Calories Per 1 Gram | Portion, Points, Serving Or Weight | Total Calories

SET MENUS *FOR* LUNCH

Name _____ Calories

Menu 1 Calorie Total

Name _____ Calories

Menu 2 Calorie Total

Name _____ Calories

Menu 3 Calorie Total

Name _____ Calories

Menu 4 Calorie Total

Name _____ Calories

Menu 5 Calorie Total

Name _____ Calories

Menu 6 Calorie Total

FOOD LIBRARY - DINNER

FOOD ITEM CALORIE CALCULATION → Calories Per 1 Gram Portion, Points, Serving Or Weight Total Calories

SET MENUS *FOR* DINNER

Name _____ Calories

Menu 1 Calorie Total

Name _____ Calories

Menu 2 Calorie Total

Name _____ Calories

Menu 3 Calorie Total

Name _____ Calories

Menu 4 Calorie Total

Name _____ Calories

Menu 5 Calorie Total

Name _____ Calories

Menu 6 Calorie Total

FOOD LIBRARY - SNACKS

FOOD ITEM	CALORIE CALCULATION	Calories Per 1 Gram	Portion, Points, Serving Or Weight	Total Calories

CALORIE LIBRARY - BEVERAGES

BEVERAGE	CALORIE CALCULATION ⟶	Cup, Glass, Can, mls OR Gram	Total Calories

Manufactured by Amazon.ca
Acheson, AB